HOW TO ACCELERATE YOUR METABOLISM?

A HEALTHY AND SUSTAINABLE WAY TO LOSE ADDI-TIONAL WEIGHT DURING A HIGH INTENSITY DIET, LOW CARB DIET AND MANY OTHER DIETS.

DAN HILD

Copyright © Dan Hild
All Rights Reserved.

ISBN 978-1-63886-472-1

This book has been published with all efforts taken to make the material error-free after the consent of the author. However, the author and the publisher do not assume and hereby disclaim any liability to any party for any loss, damage, or disruption caused by errors or omissions, whether such errors or omissions result from negligence, accident, or any other cause.

While every effort has been made to avoid any mistake or omission, this publication is being sold on the condition and understanding that neither the author nor the publishers or printers would be liable in any manner to any person by reason of any mistake or omission in this publication or for any action taken or omitted to be taken or advice rendered or accepted on the basis of this work. For any defect in printing or binding the publishers will be liable only to replace the defective copy by another copy of this work then available.

Contents

Foreword — v

1. Diets, Diets, Diets. — 1
2. Accelerating Your Metabolic Rate, The Key To Success — 3
3. Breath Your Way To A Health-ier Life — 6
4. Pu-erh Tea — 9
5. Green Coffee — 12
6. Maca Root Extract — 14
7. Good Night Drink — 16
8. Don´t Forget About Magnesium — 18
9. If It Does Not Work — 21
10. Something Worth Remembering — 22

Bibliography — 23

Disclaimer — 27

Foreword

Hello, dear reader,

If you have this book in front of you, it is very probable that you are an individual suffering with obesity. Regardless of whether it is a few kilograms or a few dozen. You have probably tried many diets, from those stating that you should eat half portions, to those consisting entirely of broths, pineapple or beats and you have noticed that going through with one of these, is, to say the least, a very difficult road.

Nevertheless, you don´t want to give up in your goal go losing weight, or wearing that shirt you loved, or simply out, you want to feel sexy and attractive again.

What I present to you in this book is not a diet with a different system, like the ones that are already in existence. And it does not matter whether you are already in a high carb diet, or a metabolic balance, or even a self-made program. The intention is to show you additional ways in which you can have more success with your diet, in order to accomplish losing more weight, without putting much more effort in it.

The secret to accomplish this is a very simple one. I will show you how to stimulate your metabolism and thus, have the ability to burn calories at a much faster rate. This book does not contain any suggestions regarding sports activity or exercise, or anything related to such topics. Not because it would not make sense to include them, but because people carrying a lot of extra weight, rarely have the ability to start and maintain such a heavy plan. First of all, because it makes them understand the limits of their bodies and their conditions, and second, because it makes the feel

FOREWORD

shame when they wonder what would people think if they saw a walrus running through the streets.

We are all acquainted with the injuries, both physical and psychological that those carrying a bit of overweight face every day. This is the reason why I would like to offer may advice to help you reach a weight in which you feel more comfortable. Of course, you should consider adding some physical activity once your mind and body allow it. But even if this is not something you wish to ponder at this moment, or in the near future, what you will find within the pages of this book will help you loose a lot of weight in a fast and efficient manner. Regardless of what diet or program you are currently on.

I wish you luck and success so you can reach your desired weight.

Yours,

Dan Hild

CHAPTER ONE

DIETS, DIETS, DIETS.

How many diets born from the products made for losing weight placed in the marked and presented through books, marketing and even complete television shows do you think there are? The answer is simple: More. Many more that you would think in your wildest dreams. And every month, you will see how a new one is born. Furthermore, there are those that already existed and are taken by somebody new, they change the name and the presentation and patent their idea.

Regardless of what your favorite diet is. This book is not made to measure their performance and give you the complete and absolute right answer.

All in all, this books is mostly about showing you that no matter what diet you have chosen, you can have a bigger rate of success by simply following some simple advices. The products here mentioned should not be considered as food supplements to be used at the same time. On the contrary: These are only products to complement your dietary plan and I invite you to know more about them. Some of them may not be recommended for you because of your diet. Some other will give you the chance to reach your desired weight faster and be able to maintain it.

Most of these advice and approaches are intended to stimulate your metabolism in order to make you reach a higher level of combustion. It is not recommendable to use all these methods at once, since the result might have a negative impact on your health because your metabolism would work at such a fast pace that it could endanger your circulation. Please, ask a professional in the field and follow the instructions given so you only take what your body could actually benefit from.2.

CHAPTER TWO

Accelerating Your Metabolic Rate, the Key to Success

wikipedia.de established the following information regarding the metabolic rate:

The metabolic rate is a variable commonly used in Zoology. It shows the energy expenditure per unit in an organism. It can calculate the output of energy that an organism presents, in calories, which can only be determined as a fraction of the energy expenditure that is released as heat.

The energy expenditure or the total revenue is understood, in the field of physiology (especially in ecophysiology) as te amount of energy per unit of time needed by a living being to maintain all processes working correctly. The energy expenditure is calculated as the base metabolism rate and the work an organism does. When it comes to estimating the work factor, it is important to consider the severity of the physical work.

HOW TO ACCELERATE YOUR METABOLISM?

The energy expenditure could be measured directly or indirectly through calories. Since the method is highly complicated, the indirect meths is used specially for larger living beings, like the human being. This is possible, thanks to the water degradation (H_2O), carbon dioxide (CO_2) and products that contain nitrogen and can be measured. From the results of said measurements the energy expenditure can be calculated with calorific values and the nutrients retained.

The energy expenditure differs, not only among species and within population, but to an individual level. During physical activity you will use much more energy than when you are resting. Furthermore, a body living in very high or very low temperatures requires more energy to maintain optimal body temperature, than one that lives in normal temperatures (see also, thermoregulation).

Within an organism, there are differences in energy expenditure as well. This is the reason why the metabolism level in the fat deposits is much less than that of organs like the heart, liver or kidney.

One can understand this quite clearly with a simple mental image:

Imagine you are in charge of keeping a very big house warm. The house owner has an agreement with local lumberjacks, who provide him with the wood they deem necessary. Since the lumberjacks would rather have a great revenue, they deliver too much, instead of too little. And every piece of wood you don´t use during the day, must be stored to avoid being stolen during the night. Your apartment is about to burst. Your new goal is to burn all the wood you were delivered during the day. If you manage to burn that wood so fast, you will be able to make room and then you would have won. You would have won more space and a much better quality of life. This is the reason why you often think of burning as much wood as possible without burning your house down or causing irreparable damage.

This is exactly the kind of things we discuss in this book. In real life, however, the lumberjacks are not the ones that are delivering the wood, but yourself who is creating reserved in your body with everything you eat at the supermarket or any other food joint. Our common goal will be, from here on, to think about the calories, which are nothing more that the energy in our food, and we will attempt to burn them as fast as we are able so your body can begin to use the reserves in your body. Only when you can manage this on a long term basis, you will have a better life quality.

CHAPTER THREE

Breath Your Way to a Health-ier Life

When I was just a child, my father would constantly tell me I was breathing the wrong way. I should do it in a deeper, more conscious way. Nowadays, I ponder that advice often. Had I only listen to him and his well-intentioned advice, instead of storing it in the know-it-all father category, I would have spared myself decades of weight issues. As well as the humiliation, the depression, the frustration and the bad habit of eating to calm my emotions.

In fact, I have recently rediscovered this concept, when a friend who is a singer talked to me about the correct way of breathing and that was after I already started losing weight.

She simply asked me how I managed to lose such a big amount of weight, since she had lost around twenty kilograms when she was just beginning her studies. Only now she realizes that a breathing deeply greatly accelerates your metabolism and makes the extra weight, practically vanish by itself.

The fact is that the cells that are not absorbing enough oxygen o for some other reason, do not receive the necessary amount, are not performing their tasks like they should. Surviving is the goal and this is not the best way to perform up to the tasks. This is the way cells work in nature: combustion requires oxygen, and when the cells get too little of it, they just light up, but they don´t burn.

The result comes in two ways: First, the body consumes less energy, thus calories. Plus, the cell does not manage to carry its task adequately. This happens, regardless of these cells pertaining to the heart, the kidney, the brain, or the nervous system. They simply do not work like they are intended. Many researchers believe that receiving low oxygen amounts has an effect on the fact that people age prematurely, or even in diseases such as cancer. Otto Warburg received the Nobel Prize in 1931 and was appropriately honored for his accomplishments in this field by the Federal Republic of Germany with his own postmark[1].

Taking into account that we wish to accelerate the metabolism, here you will find an exercise which should be carried on three times a day, in sessions of five minutes each. The three steps, are the following:

- Inhale deeply with your stomach through your nose while you count to five in your head.

- Now, hold the air within your body and at the same speed, count from 0, to 15.

- Finally, exhale through your mouth while you count to eight.

This exercise should be carried on 10 to 12 times, per session. You will notice that after a few days of doing it, you will have more energy. If you add this exercise to a diet program, you will notice success will come much faster.

You will notice quite fast that that tiredness that comes after each meal, is less every time. The reason for this fatigue in most cases, is not because the body is full, but rather to the fact that the heart has been working for a half-day and has used up a lot of oxygen, and that makes him lose strength through the decrease of oxygen in the blood. Once the remaining oxygen is used for the digestive process, there is still less for the heart to function properly. This is why, the body, attempting to protect itself enters into a resting mode. Nevertheless, if you perform these breathing exercises in the morning, and at noon, there will be enough oxygen for digesting and for the heart to function properly, letting your body remain powerful.

[1]*wikipedia.es*:
Otto Heinrich Warburg (Freiburg, October 8, 1883 - Berlin, August 1, 1970) was a german physiologist. In 1931 he was congratulated with the Nobel Prize for Physiology or Medicine, for his "discovery of nature and the method of action of the respiratory enzyme."

CHAPTER FOUR

PU-ERH TEA

Pu-Erh tea is derived from the same plant as common black tea, but it´s different from it, because it´s produced in a different way.

This different method of production means that tea has a variety of ingredients, which degrade very much in the process that black tea requires. There is a very interesting presentation about this tea, published recently by Peter Carl Simons.

While in Germany, the German Nutrition Society (DGE, acronym in German) warns about this tea, it has been used successfully for many centuries in its country of origin as part of traditional medicine in China. Furthermore, it has been discovered and exposed more and more in many well-known universities across the United States and Europe.

The Pu-Ehr Tea is normally presented as a product for losing weight. Without providing any scientific evidence, the German Nutrition Society has established that this is not the case. Furthermore, they have warned about its contents y since it contains stimulant substances such as caffeine and theobromine that could pose harm if they the Pu-Ehr tea is consumed in excess.

Caffeine, as I am sure you are aware of, is what your coffee contains and theobromine is the substance that makes 1 to 2.5% of the cocoa beans originated from the cocoa tree. We can also find it in the common cola beverage, mate, or black tea. Back chocolate contains amounts from 3 to 10 g of theobromine pero kilogram, depending on the company that makes it. Certainly, the DGE, is right about these substances should not be consumed in excess, but we would then have to add milk, cheese, wine, herb and mint tea to that list.

Many clinical trials and tests have proven that Pu-Ehr tea does not only manage to accelerate the metabolic level in a significant way, thus stimulating the burning of fat, but also has positive effects on the immune system, reduces cholesterol and fat levels in your blood.

Pu-Ehr tea is the, a wonderful support to any diet. Consumed moderately, this tea accelerates your metabolism in a perfect way. Experts state that the maximum amount to consume per day should be 1 to 2 liters.

As for storing and preparing it, Simons writes in his book:

Whether you wish to drink the Pu-Ehr tea for health reasons or only to enjoy it: it is important you store your tea correctly. Please, take into account that Pu-Ehr tea is fermented naturally, and while it rests in your kitchen, it may continue to evolve. This is the reason why it should not be stored in a place without proper ventilation. The ideal recipient would be a ceramic vase without detailing.

The difference between this one and there teas, is that Pu-Ehr tea can be stored for a long time. In China, ancient teas from different varieties are offered. This could be compared to the offer for wine that exists in the market. You could find tea that has been stored for over 50 years in the market. If stored correctly, these could gain nutrients and a better taste with the passing of time. High-quality products can be stored for much longer and these varieties can be as expensive as high quality wines.

If you bought your tea in a recipient, you should remove the leaves with a sharp object and with extreme care. In China, a special kind of knife is used for this tea. With the fine blade, you can remove the leaves from the container, without damaging or breaking them. Broken leaves give you a sour taste. Tea connoisseurs use a typical Chinese pot made out of clay to prepare it. Those who do not own this kind of pot, can use a common teapot.

Then, you add 5 to 20 grams of leaves to the pot and fill it with 1/4 of boiling water, depending on the quality of the tea. The first infusion is poured a few seconds later, but it should not be consumed, because of its strength and sourness. Only from the second infusion on, should it be enjoyable. The already humid leaves are covered in boiling water. After five to ten-seconds, you can pour the tea into another recipient. The soaked leaves can be used for another five to ten infusions. But, the taste and quality of the ingredients is better during the first five infusions, (the first one, the strong and sour one, does not count).

Tea is consumed slowly and in small sips.

CHAPTER FIVE

GREEN COFFEE

A wonderful and alternate option to Pu-Erh tea is green coffee. Green coffee is not meant as immature coffee or organic tea. It actually inly refers to the coffee beans when they have not yet been roasted. This is the natural product, and every day, the number of individuals that roast coffee by themselves, through an appliance they buy, is bigger.

This has a lot to do with the fact that green coffee is easier to get and more available every time in central and south America, as well as in Africa, in half a kilogram or a whole kilogram packages.

Green coffee, compared to conventional coffee contains significantly higher levels of vitamins, since many of the nutrients and good substances in it, are destroyed in the roasting process. And, regarding its use during a diet, or as a supplement, it is useful because of it contains a high level of chlorogenic acid.

wikipedia.de states:

Chlorogenic acid is a known antioxidant and its isomers protect the DNA from any kind of harm, with effects that have given good results in such extreme cases as those of cells harmed by radioactive radiation. After the body receives food, it reduces the absorption of sugar in the bloodstream.

This supports the theory that chlorogenic acid shows an anti-diabetic effect in living beings. Furthermore, in individuals with good health, it reduces blood pressure. Chlorogenic acid stops the blood from coagulating. And in studies, performed in Switzerland, with mice as the subject, it showed to have a positive effect in multiple kinds of gastric ulcers, as well as its ability to stop liver inflammation. Finally, it has been proven that chlorogenic acid can activate the programmed death of cancer cells.

With more detail, Peter Carl Simmons states in his book :

During the process of burning fat, chlorogenic acid is especially important. It is the base of the fat burning effects of green coffee. During the roasting of coffee beans, these nutrients and effects are greatly destroyed.

A simplified way to look at it is to sat that chlorogenic acid stops the absorption and storing of sugar in the body. And if the body starts absorbing less sugar, it automatically reduces fat, since the body starts to work with the fat it has stored in it. The result of a constant use of green coffee manages to decreases the levels of body fat, and thus, reduces weight.

CHAPTER SIX

Maca Root Extract

The maca root extract is an important source of energy which brings life to a body, especially in the morning and it also accelerates the metabolism.

The maca root extract grows in its origin country, in the Peruvian Andes at a 3,800 to 4,800 elevation over sea level. Regardless of these inadequate conditions and in combination with the air, this plant manages to absorb every nutrient available for it in its root. For the natives this is an important source of nourishment, which proves that one is not able to overdose on its use.

Mainly, maca root extract is used to treat erectile disfunction, as well as hormonal problems or infertility in women. Furthermore, maca is used by bodybuilders as a natural alternative to steroids. This is the reason why it is widely available around the world.

When it comes to a diet, two of the effects of the maca can cause great interest. First, it helps in the forming of muscles. Of course, this may cause a negative bad impression when one is trying to lose weight, because the more muscles mass you get, the more weight you put on.

But this would be a failed approach since every muscular fiber burns calories during day and night, and if we are talking long-term, this would be the perfect support to our dietary problem.

Just as important, the maca root gives you a boost of energy. The black root is the most successful when it comes to this. There are also red and yellow roots. In my case, taking 500 to 1,000 milligrams of maca root in the mornings, works much better than the strongest coffee. Furthermore, the metabolism gets stimulated and as described by Simmons, it keeps us in a good mood and guarantees us a good day.

CHAPTER SEVEN

GOOD NIGHT DRINK

Many diet programs, and especially those in magazines dramatically lower the intake of protein during a diet. These are theories that should never be used anymore. Since many years ago it has been known that the lack of protein in a diet is the most common cause if gaining the weight all over. In fact, the main objective of any diet should be to maintain a good amount of muscle and offer the body the appropriate amount of protein. Scientific studies show that 2 grams per kilogram should suffice. A person that weights 90 kilograms, would need 180 grams to keep the existing muscles and at the very same time, cover the additional need for protein the body has.

What the creators of low protein diets don´t know or choose to deliberately ignore is that every arm of muscle is burning fat every second, whether we are moving or even asleep. And while it is true that this mass weights, it is also true that it helps us reduce weight, and maintain a healthy ratio of fat burning. An approach such as that of a low protein diet is as bad of an idea as a car thinking that the weight of the car is reducing its speed and decides to get rid of its most important part, the engine.

The recommended amount of protein may sound exaggerated, but f we take into account the fact that every second around 50 million cells are replaces by new ones in the human body, and proteins represent the biggest component of those cells, then we can understand we are not exaggerating.

An old and dear friend told me a few years ago about this Good Night Drink, and I must admit, I was skeptical at first. Nevertheless, I decided to give it a try. The mix is very simple:

- 40g of protein powder (with a quality CFM, if possible)
- 1 teaspoon of honey
- freshly squeezed lemon juice (organic)
- 0.3 to 0.5 liters of fresh water

Every ingredient is mixed and drunk an hour before going to sleep. My experience has been the following:

- After years having problems to sleep, I now sleep wonderfully.
- The lemon juice stimulates my metabolism even during the night, I burn more calories and I have a better digestion.
- High quality protein makes sure my body gets the much needed worries in its state to keep performing in an optimal way and make sure there is no loss in muscle mass.

CHAPTER EIGHT

Don´t forget about Magnesium

Many people nowadays suffer from a strong magnesium deficiency. Nevertheless, many do not notice. There are plenty of reasons for this:

Our food contains less minerals

- We eat less leafy vegetables and whole grains, where a lot of magnesium could be acquired.
- Drinks with phosphate, such as cola beverages, reduce the intake of magnesium.
- Even when drinking small amounts of alcohol, an approximate of 50 mg of magnesium is excreted by the kidneys.
- Magnesium helps our body to better handle any kind of stress or tension, but needs enormous amounts of it to accomplish it.

Then, why do we need magnesium for? The answer to this question is not so simple. Magnesium is somewhat the manager of 3,000 enzymes in our body. This affects a considerable variety of physical processes. Many books, particularly the book Minerals, the successful program by Strung and Jopp, show these relationships in a much better way. Even when we can find much more detailed information in the book, you can grasp the main idea about the benefits of magnesium by just reading the titles of the chapters it contains :

- Magnesium against stress
- Sleep better
- The Good Mood Shower during PMS
- A relaxed pregnancy
- 1 out of 10 Germans uses magnesium against migraine
- Magnesium, the source of energy for athletes
- Burn fat faster during aerobics
- Can Magnesium protect you against diabetes?
- Lower the risk of a heart attack

Most people would find all these very useful. And if that was not the case, at least one of these would call for your attention. When the goal is losing weight, there are two aspects to consider:

One, in order to lose weight, sleeping is crucial. And it is much more important than you would think, since many studies state that in many cases, sleeping poor is one of the biggest reasons for obesity.

Magnesium has always been mentioned when it comes to getting a good quality sleep. First of all, magnesium calms the nerves, which also helps fighting stress. Another common reason why people sleep poorly is because of tense muscles. Magnesium acts very quickly against tired legs and cramps. And since it also helps reducing blood pressure, it helps you sleep.

In order to work properly, cells need magnesium. This affects the cells responsible for your digestion as well as those in charge of nourishing your muscles, including once again your heart. Here we can prove once more what has already been discussed about breathing and oxygen. A magnesium deficiency causes the mitochondria which is considered the source of energy of the cells, to lose power. Less power, means burning less and less combustion, means less calorie burning.

Experts advice to take 200 milligrams of magnesium an hour before going to sleep. It is also recommended to take the same amount every morning. Depending on your daily routine, whether that means a sports activity, stress, or any other reason, you could take a higher dose.

CHAPTER NINE

IF IT DOES NOT WORK

Many people have reasons for their weight problems that do not always present themselves as a physical problem o for eating poorly. Many people, whether they are conscious or not, gain weight to calm the pain, to punish themselves or others, protect themselves, or for many other reasons.

It is clear that these problems cannot be solved by lowering the intake of calories o burning more calories. One of the first persons to address this issue in his books and shed light on how to get through them, is Christoph Bisel, from BMI Coach GmbH . In his book, "I was a Beached Whale: How I lost more than 60 pounds - fast and efficiently - and this is how you can do it too!,"[1] he describes his own experience dealing with weight problems and the bases of his approach as a health coach.

[1] Bisel, Christoph: I was a Beached Whale: How I lost more than 60 pounds - fast and efficiently - and this is how you can do it too!, CreateSpace, 2015

CHAPTER TEN

SOMETHING WORTH REMEMBERING

Everything stated in this book is based in personal experiences, my clients´ experiences or in the many studies carried on around the world. This is why is necessary to consult a health professional, before taking any advice along with your diet program. The information presented here should not replace the professional opinion of a health professional, or there recommendations, and / or dosage. Every single body reacts differently. Obviously, not everything this book contains should be considered as a promise of salvation.

Bibliography

- Barcroft, Alasdair: Aloe Vera: Nature's Silent Healer, 2003, Baam
- Bankhofer, Prof. Hademar: Aloe Vera - Die Pflanze für Gesundheit, Vitalität und Wohlbefinden, 2013, Kneipp Verlag, 6. Auflage
- Beringer, Alice: Aloe vera - Die Königin der Heilpflanzen: Natürlich gesund und schön durch den reinen Extrakt der Aloe vera, 2007, Heyne
- Dahlke, Rüdiger: Krankheit als Symbol, 2014, C. Bertelsmann, 22. Auflage
- Dahlke, Rüdiger: Gewichtsprobleme, 1989, Knaur
- Delbé, Jean B.: Gesund werden - gesund bleiben: Aloe-Vera-Leitfaden Gesund bleiben, 2004, M+M Verlag
- Finnegan, John &, Schmid, Rainer: Aloe Vera - das Geschenk der Natur an uns alle, 2014, Ernährung & Gesundheit, 35. Auflage
- Fricke, Dr. Ulrich (Hrsg.): Heilen mit Vitalstoffen, 2008, FID
- Frauwallner, Anita: Was tun, wenn der Darm streikt?, 2012, Kneipp
- Gray, Robert: Das Darmheilungsbuch, 2011, Trias
- Grout, Pam: Atme dich schlank, 2014, Ullstein
- Hendel, Dr. Barbara. Das Magnesium Buch, 2014, VAK
- Hild, Anne: Die hcg Diät, 2014, Aurum, 11. Auflage
- Jünemann, Matthias: Die Adipositas Kur, 2012, BOD, 2. Auflage
- Kraske, Dr. med. Eva-Maria: Säure-Basen Balance, 2005, Gräfe & Unzer
- Oppermann, Jutta: Aloe Vera - Was die Pflanze wirklich

BIBLIOGRAPHY

- kann, 2004, Lebensbaum
- Peuser, Michael: Kapillaren bestimmen unser Schicksal: Aloe - Kaiserin der Heilpflanzen, Quelle für Vitalität und Gesundheit, 2010, St. Hubertus
- Rahn-Huber, Ulla: Natürlich heilen und pflegen mit Aloe vera, 2015, Riwei
- Schikowsky, Arno; Binder, Dr. med. Rudolf; Mörwald, Christian: Die 21-Tage Stoffwechselkur, 2014
- Simons, Peter Carl: Chlorophyll - Gesundheit ist grün, 2015, BOD
- Simons, Peter Carl: Grüner Kaffee - die Garantie zum Abnehmen, 2015, BOD
- Simons, Peter Carl: Aloe Vera - 6'000 Jahre Medizingeschichte können sich nicht irren, 2015, BOD
- Simons, Peter Carl: Pu-Erh-Tee - Tee der Kaiser, 2015, BOD
- Simons, Peter Carl: Maca - Die Heilpflanze der Inkas, 2015, BOD
- Skinner, Rosalynd: Aloe Vera: The Medicine Plant, 2005, Mill Enterprises
- Skousen, Max B.: Aloe Vera Handbook: The Ancient Egyptian Medicine Plant, 2005, Book Publishing Company
- Strunz, Dr. Ulrich, Jopp, Andreas: Forever Young Geheimnis Eiweiss, 2013, Heyne, 7. Auflage
- Strunz, Dr. Ulrich, Jopp, Andreas: Mineralien - das Erfolgsprogramm, 2012, Heyne, 5. Auflage
- Treutwein, Norbert: Übersäuerung - Krank ohne Grund;1996, Südwest Verlag
- Wu, Dr. Li: Fatburner Pu-Erh-Tee, 1999, Midena (Weltbild)
- Vollmer, Joachim Bernd: Gesunder Darm, gesundes Leben, 2010, Knaur

BIBLIOGRAPHY

- Zittlau, Dr. Jörg: Grüner Tee für Gesundheit und Vitalität, 1997, Ludwig

Disclaimer

Introduction

By using this book, you accept this disclaimer in full.

No advice

The book contains information. The information is not advice, and should not be treated as such.

If you think you may be suffering from any medical condition you should seek immediate medical attention. You should never delay seeking medical advice, disregard medical advice, or discontinue medical treatment because of information in the book.

No representations or warranties

To the maximum extent permitted by applicable law and subject to section below, we exclude all representations, warranties, undertakings and guarantees relating to the book.

Without prejudice to the generality of the foregoing paragraph, we do not represent, warrant, undertake or guarantee:

- that the information in the book is correct, accurate, complete or non-misleading;

- that the use of the guidance in the book will lead to any particular outcome or result.

Limitations and exclusions of liability

The limitations and exclusions of liability set out in this section and elsewhere in this disclaimer: are subject to section 6 below; and govern all liabilities arising under the disclaimer or in relation to the book, including liabilities arising in contract, in tort (including negligence) and for breach of statutory duty.

We will not be liable to you in respect of any losses arising out of any event or events beyond our reasonable control.

We will not be liable to you in respect of any business losses, including without limitation loss of or damage to profits, income, revenue, use, production, anticipated savings, business, contracts, commercial opportunities or goodwill.

We will not be liable to you in respect of any loss or corruption of any data, database or software.

We will not be liable to you in respect of any special, indirect or consequential loss or damage.

Exceptions

Nothing in this disclaimer shall: limit or exclude our liability for death or personal injury resulting from negligence; limit or exclude our liability for fraud or fraudulent misrepresentation; limit any of our liabilities in any way that is not permitted under applicable law; or exclude any of our liabilities that may not be excluded under applicable law.

Severability

If a section of this disclaimer is determined by any court or other competent authority to be unlawful and/or unenforceable, the other sections of this disclaimer continue in effect.

If any unlawful and/or unenforceable section would be lawful or enforceable if part of it were deleted, that part will be deemed to be deleted, and the rest of the section will continue in effect.

Law and jurisdiction

DISCLAIMER

This disclaimer will be governed by and construed in accordance with Swiss law, and any disputes relating to this disclaimer will be subject to the exclusive jurisdiction of the courts of Switzerland.

www.ingramcontent.com/pod-product-compliance
Lightning Source LLC
Chambersburg PA
CBHW020714180526
45163CB00008B/3087